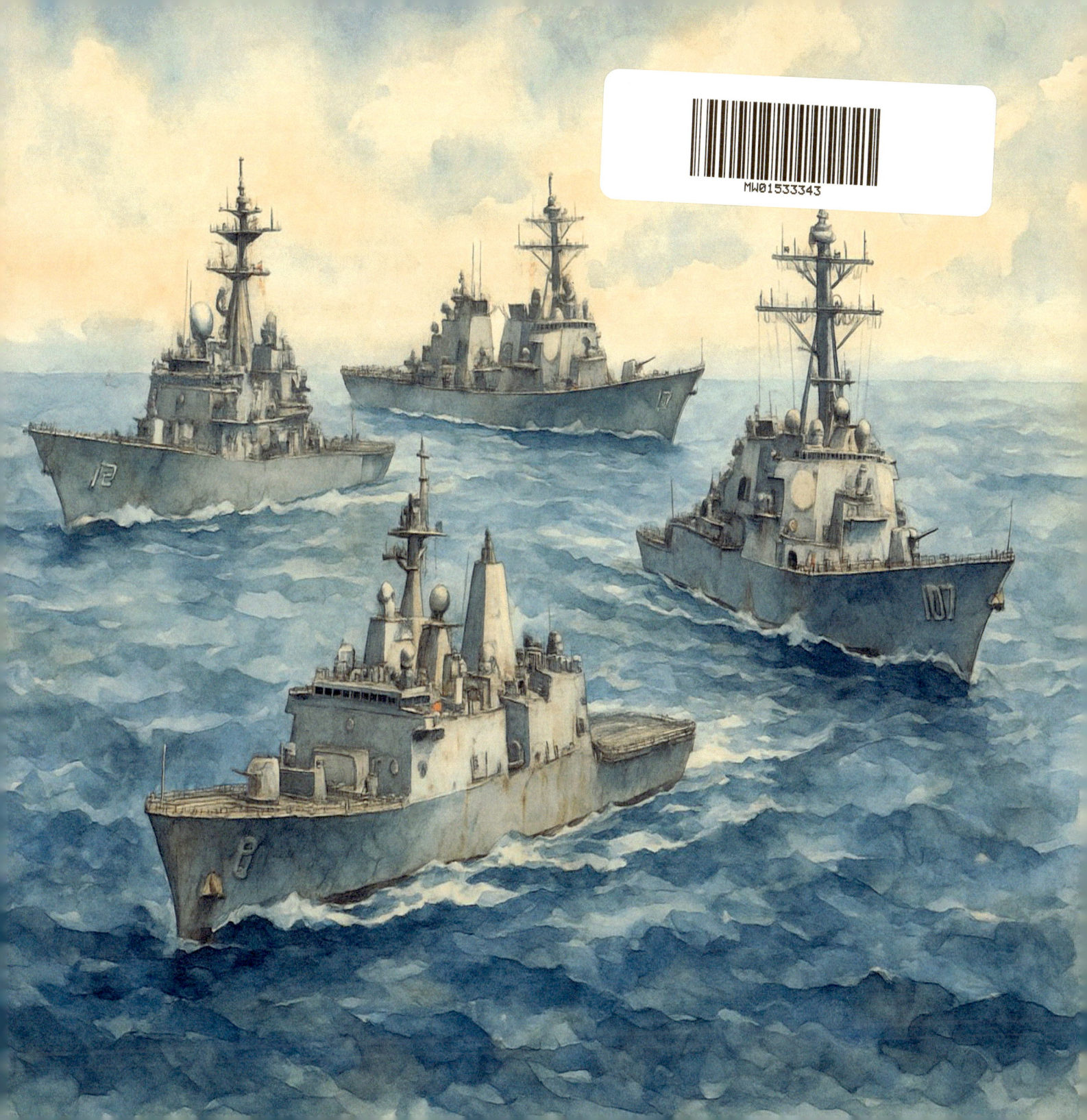

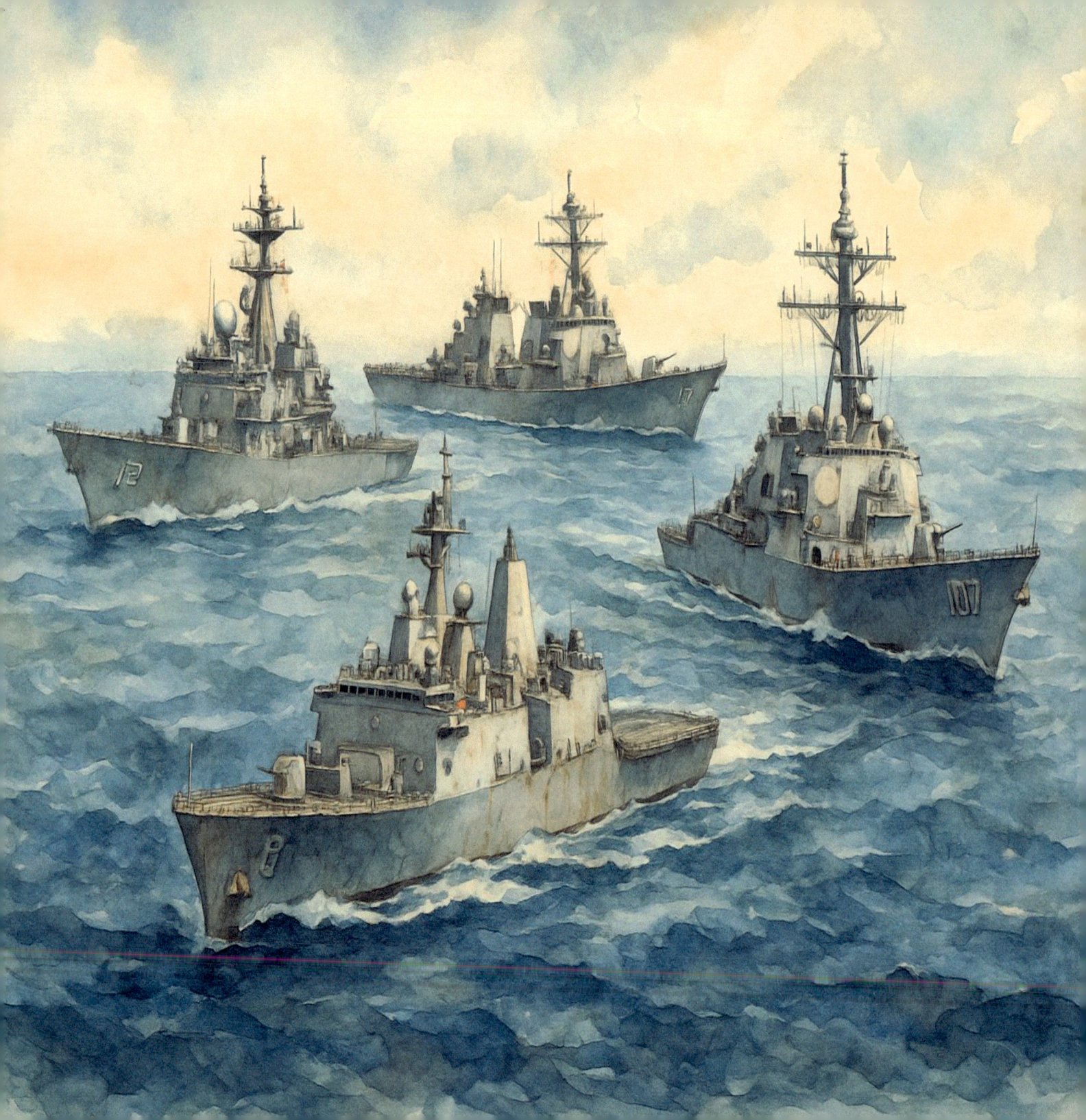

Boots, Boats, and Hugs That Last

Nicky and Eleni

My sweet dandelion children,

Military life can be hard, but may this book be a warm light for you on the days that feel the darkest. Always remember how deeply you are loved.

I love you forever,

Mom

To all the military kids—the dandelion children—you are deeply loved and never alone.

To the parents reading this, you are doing better than you think.

Some days may feel hard, like you're just getting by, but you are not failing.

You're raising incredible kids who are growing up strong in a world that's anything but "normal."

I see you. I support you. And you are enough.

Remember to breathe, to feel, and to let your heart speak.

You are brave, amazing, and more resilient than you know.

Keep going—you're doing an incredible job.

And remember, no matter the distance or the days ahead, love always finds its way back home.

Dr. Julia A. Priftis
Military Spouse and Mother

My name is Nicky, I'm five and a half,
I burp the ABCs and make people laugh.
I skip-count by twos and I'm super-duper fast,
Except when I'm tying my sneakers... at last.

My dad's in the Navy - he works on a ship,
With helmets and walkie-talkies
and tools on his hip.
He wears giant boots
and a hat with a flap,
And sometimes he
falls asleep right
in time for a nap!
He sails on the
ocean with sailors
and snacks,
And calls me from
places that don't
show on maps.

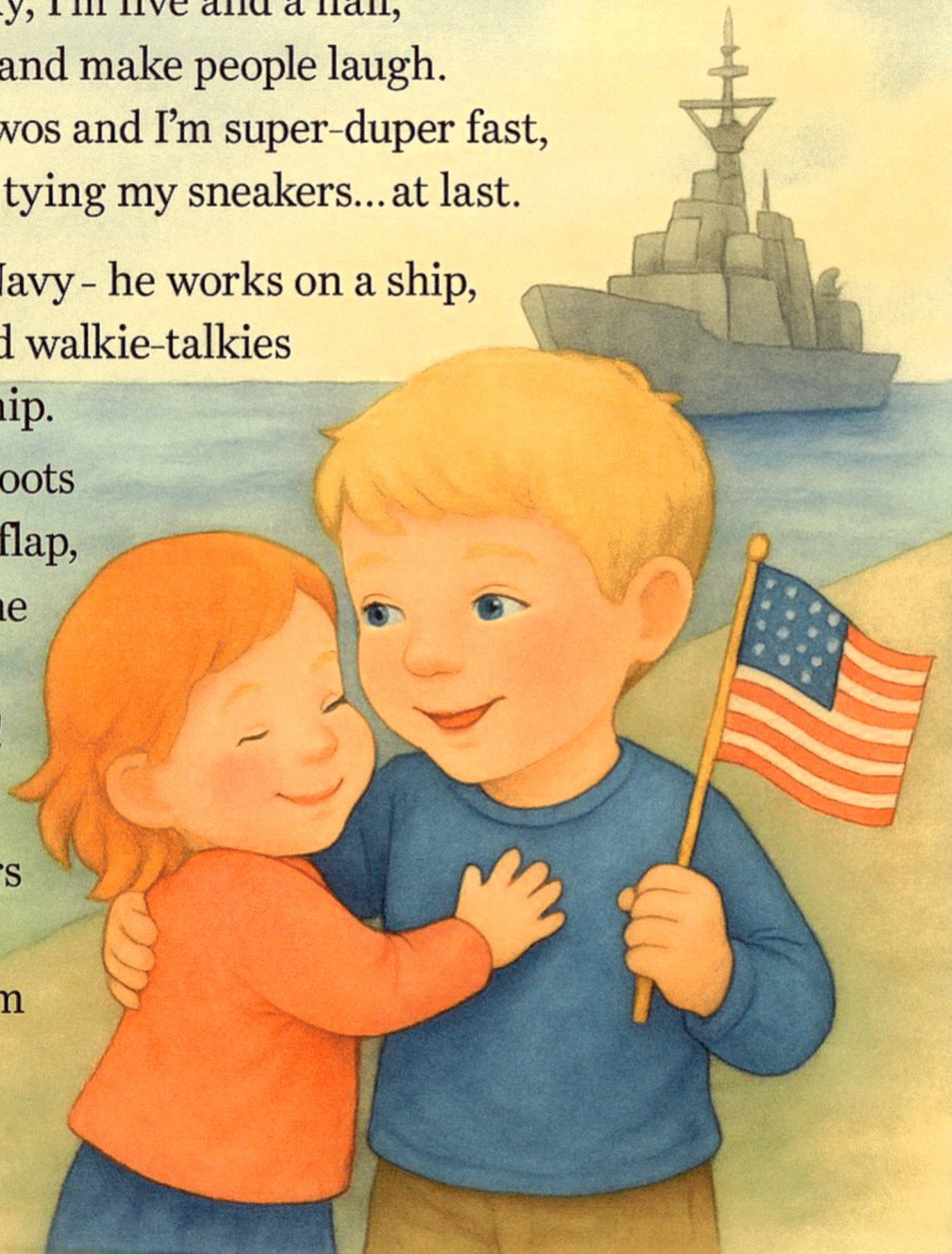

He's helping folks, all brave and bold,
With stories I'll hear when I'm big and old.
He packs his bag with snacks and gear,
I add a note and zip it up clear!

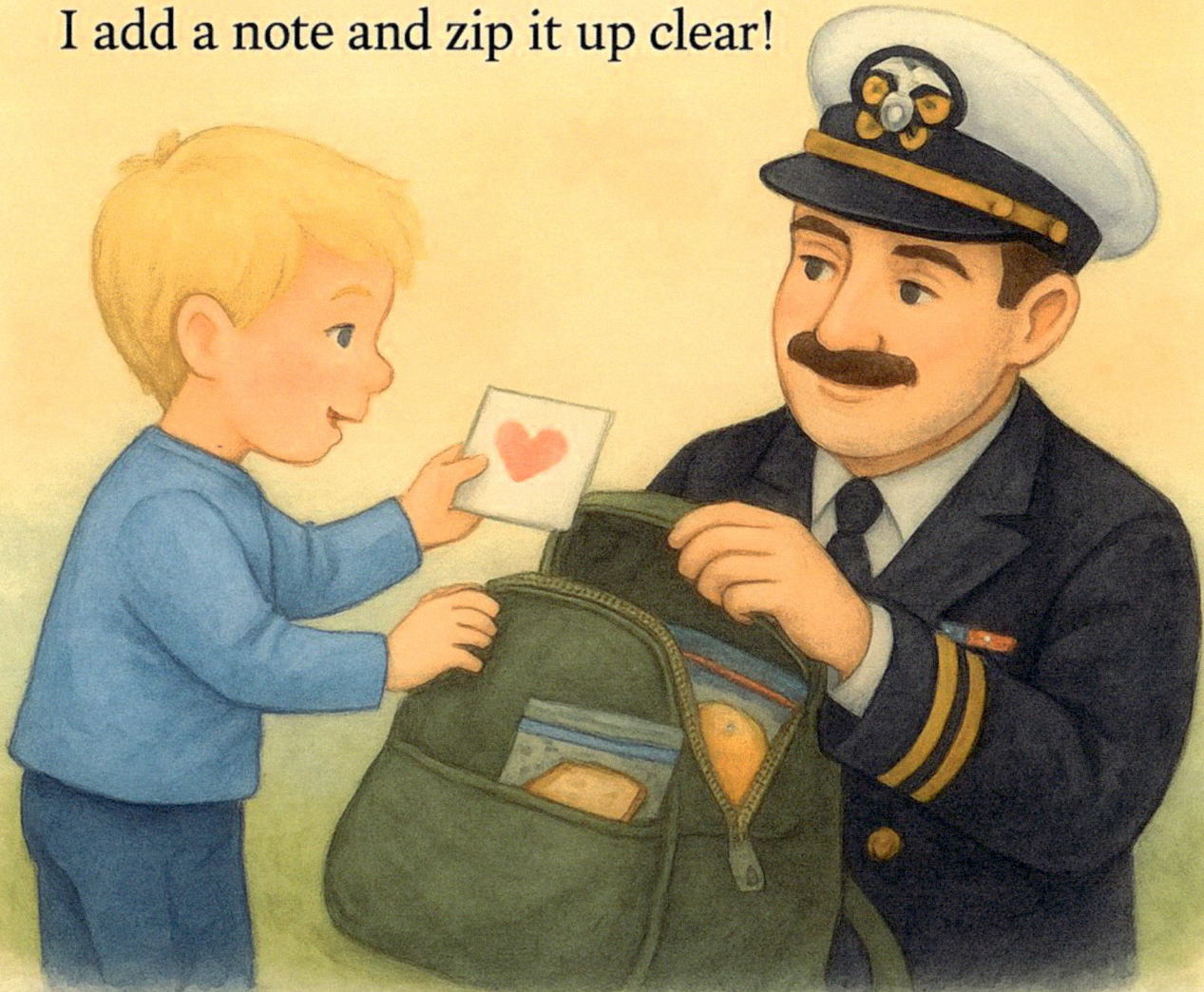

Sometimes he goes to places far, far away,
Where the sun might play or the clouds might stay.
He calls it deployment —I call it a trip,
On a big, splashy ship —not a boat with a slip!

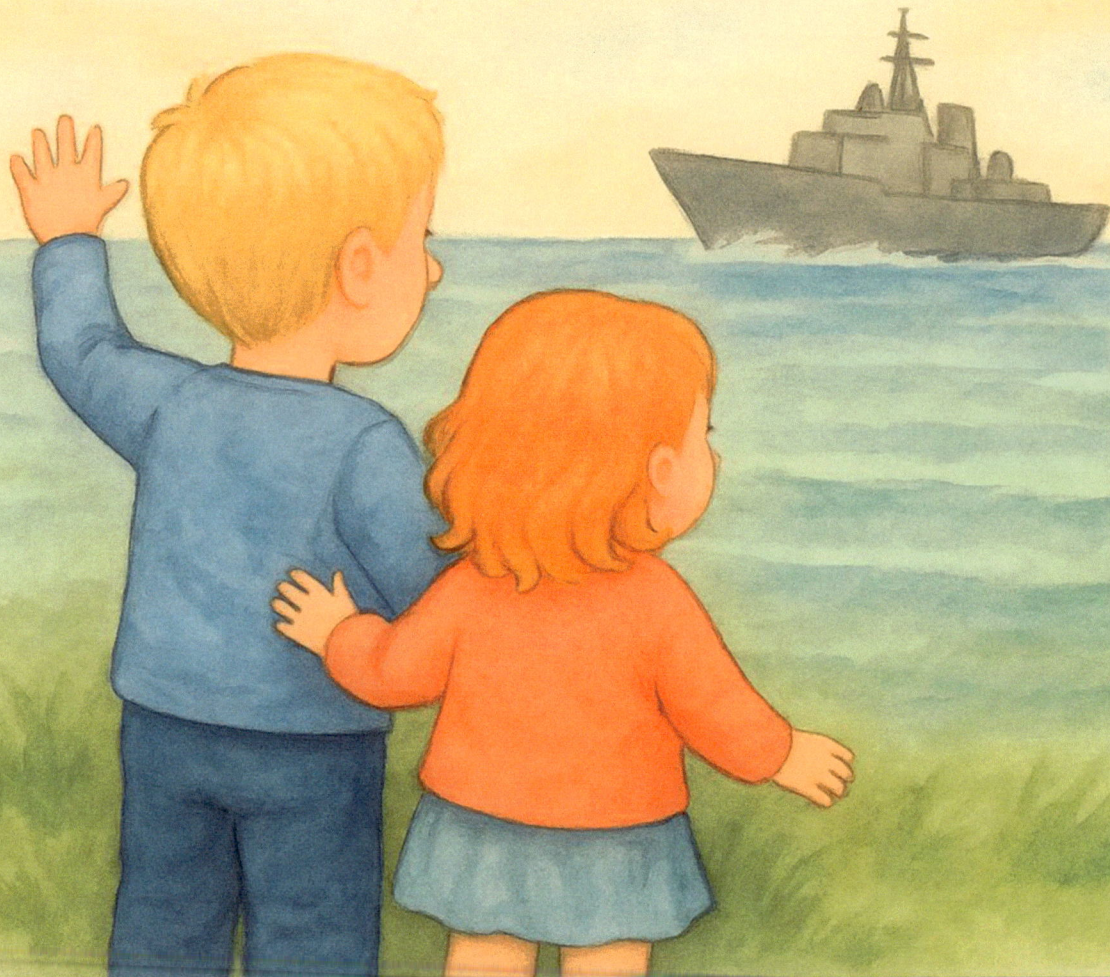

We make a paper chain, all shiny and bright,
We call them 'Love You Loops'–they're a silly delight!
Each day I snip one with a big, goofy grin,
Counting down the days 'til Dad's home again!

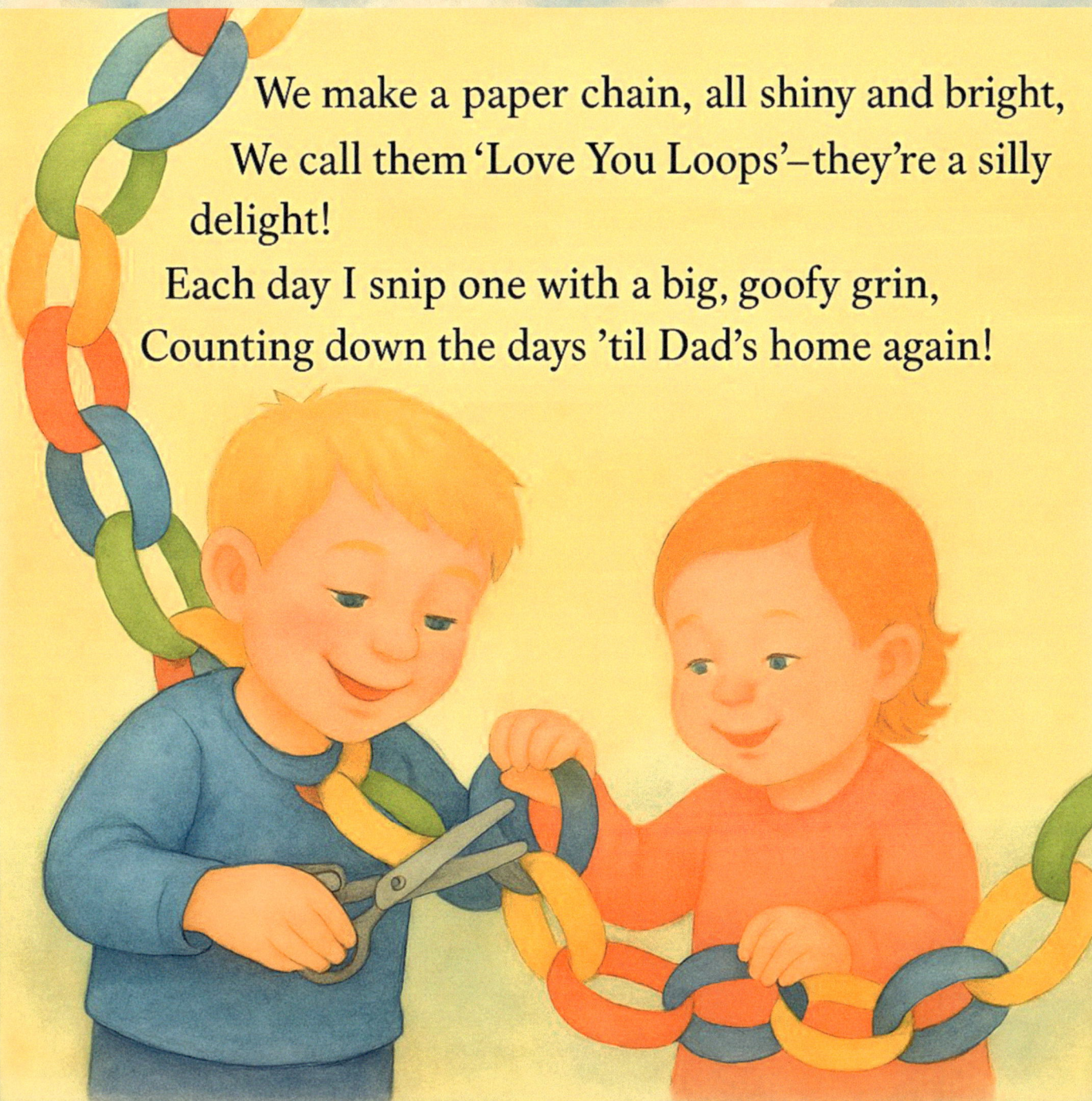

When Daddy leaves, I feel quite small,
Like I might cry or hug my Daddy doll-

Sometimes I smile, then feel bad too—
What if Daddy feels sad too?

So I draw pictures, bold and bright,
And pack them in a box just right!

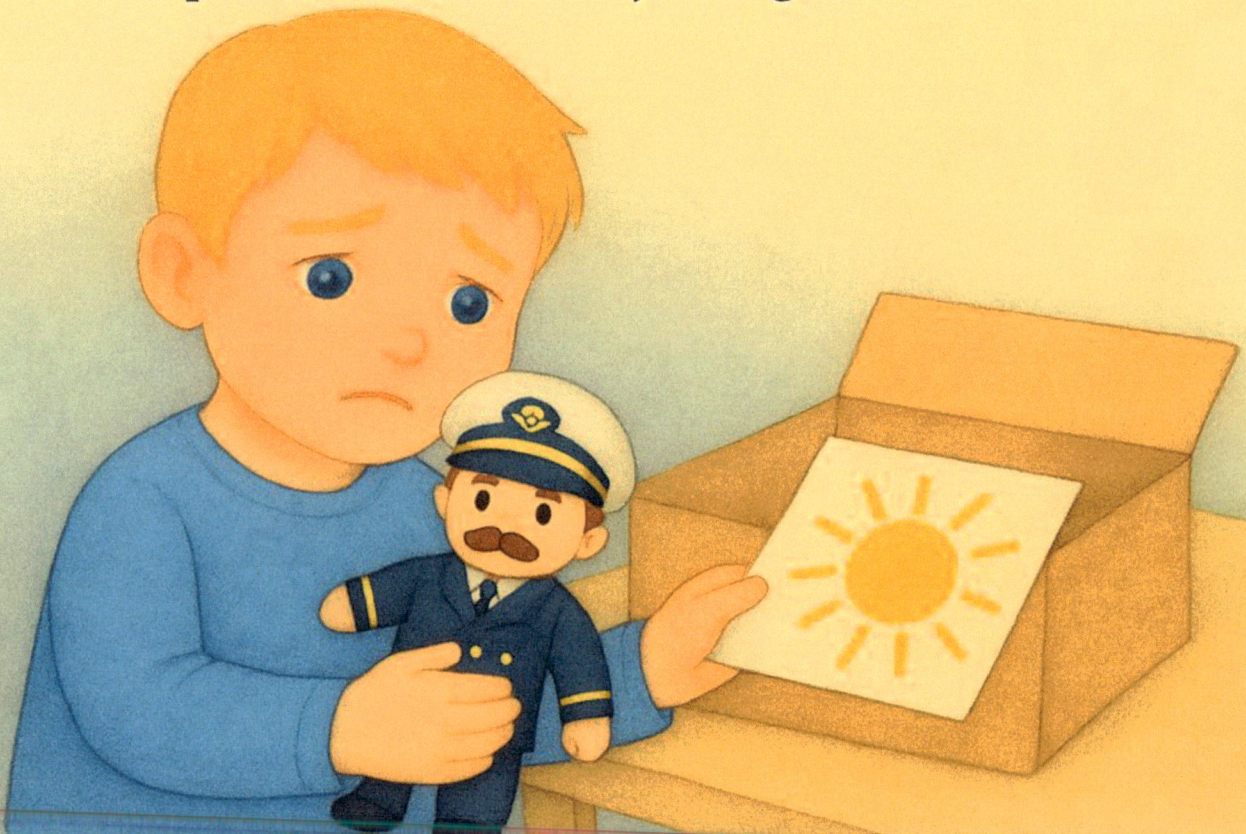

Sometimes my feelings go splash and then swirl,
Like riding big waves in a crazy sea whirl!
I'm happy, then sad, then mad, then glad—
"Is this normal?" I ask. "Yep! Being a military kid,
I'm rad!"

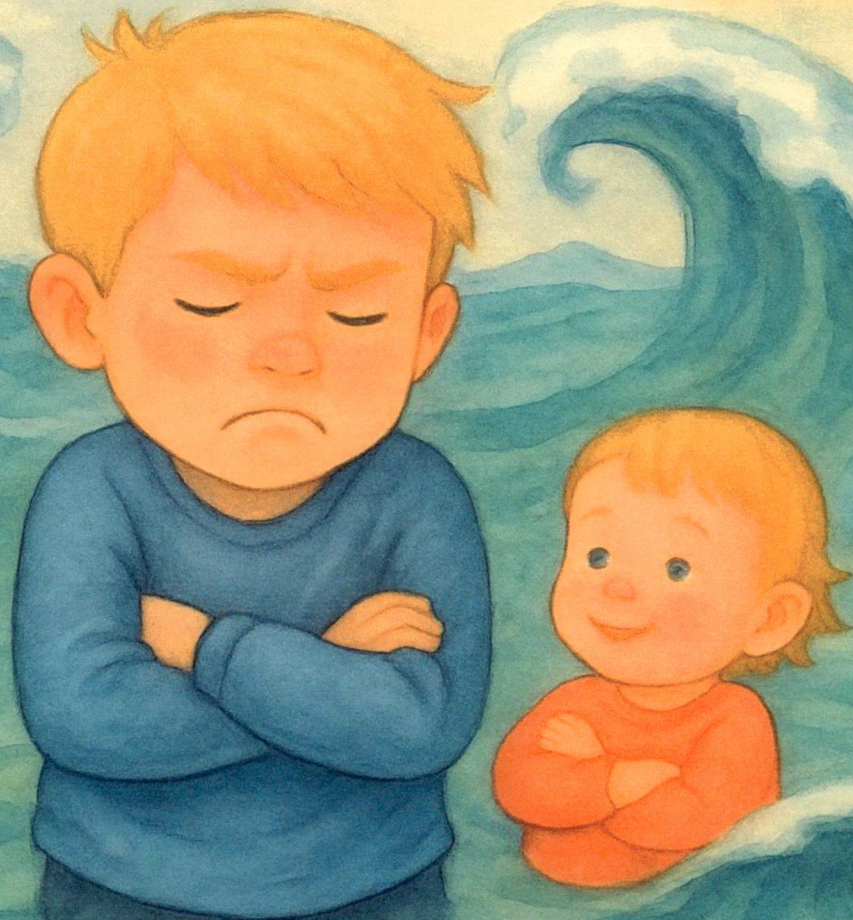

Mom says, 'Yes!' with a wink and a grin,
We do a Feeling Check-In—let the fun begin!
'Today I'm dark,' I sometimes say loud,
Then other times, 'I'm excited!'
and jump like a cloud.

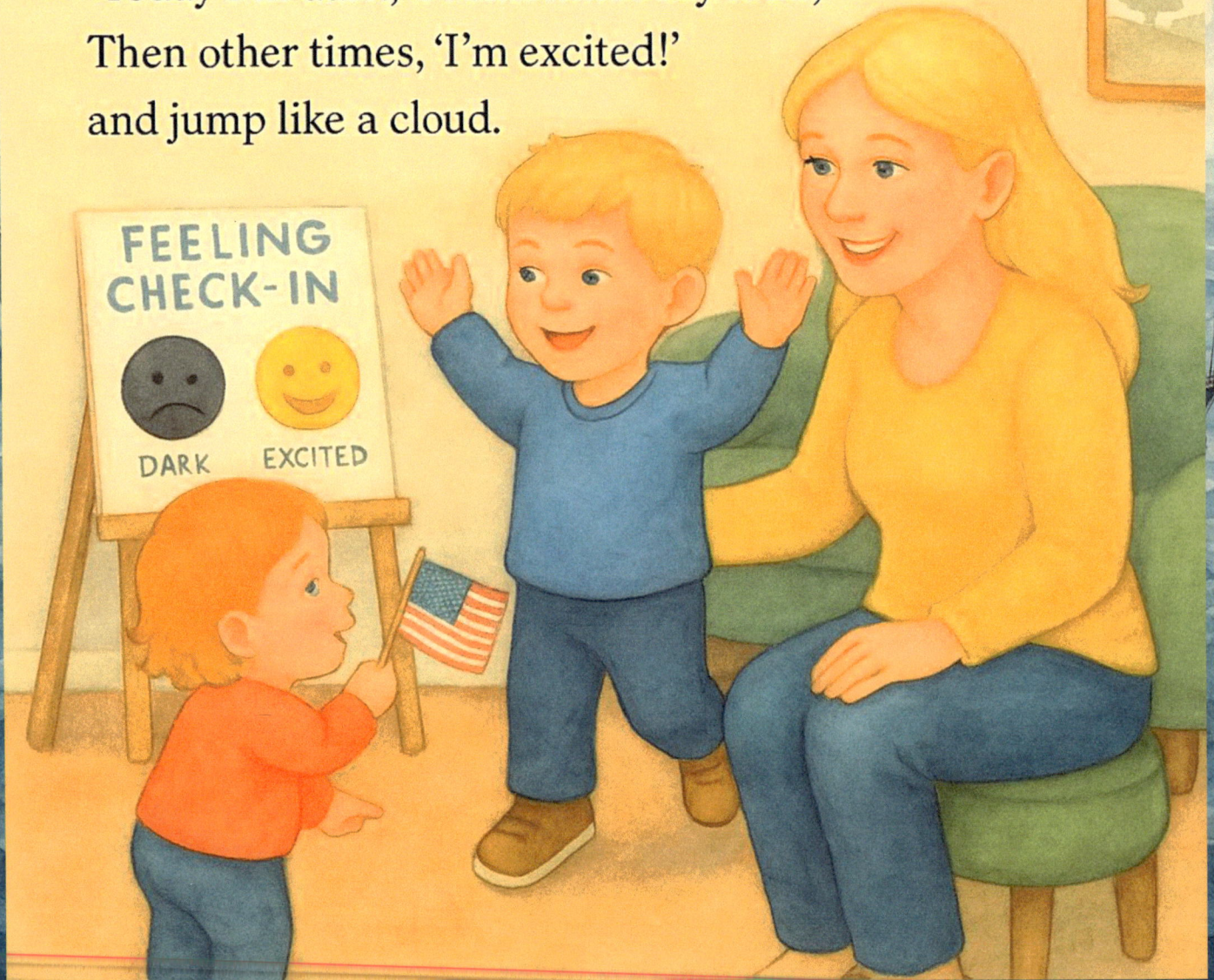

FEELING
CHECK-IN

DARK   EXCITED

When Daddy's away, we send him surprise boxes,
Filled with drawings of flowers and big, noisy foxes.
I once sent a cat trying hard to climb trees,
And lots of goofy jokes—including 'fart sneeze!'
I always make sure to send him a smile,
So he knows I'm thinking of him all the while!

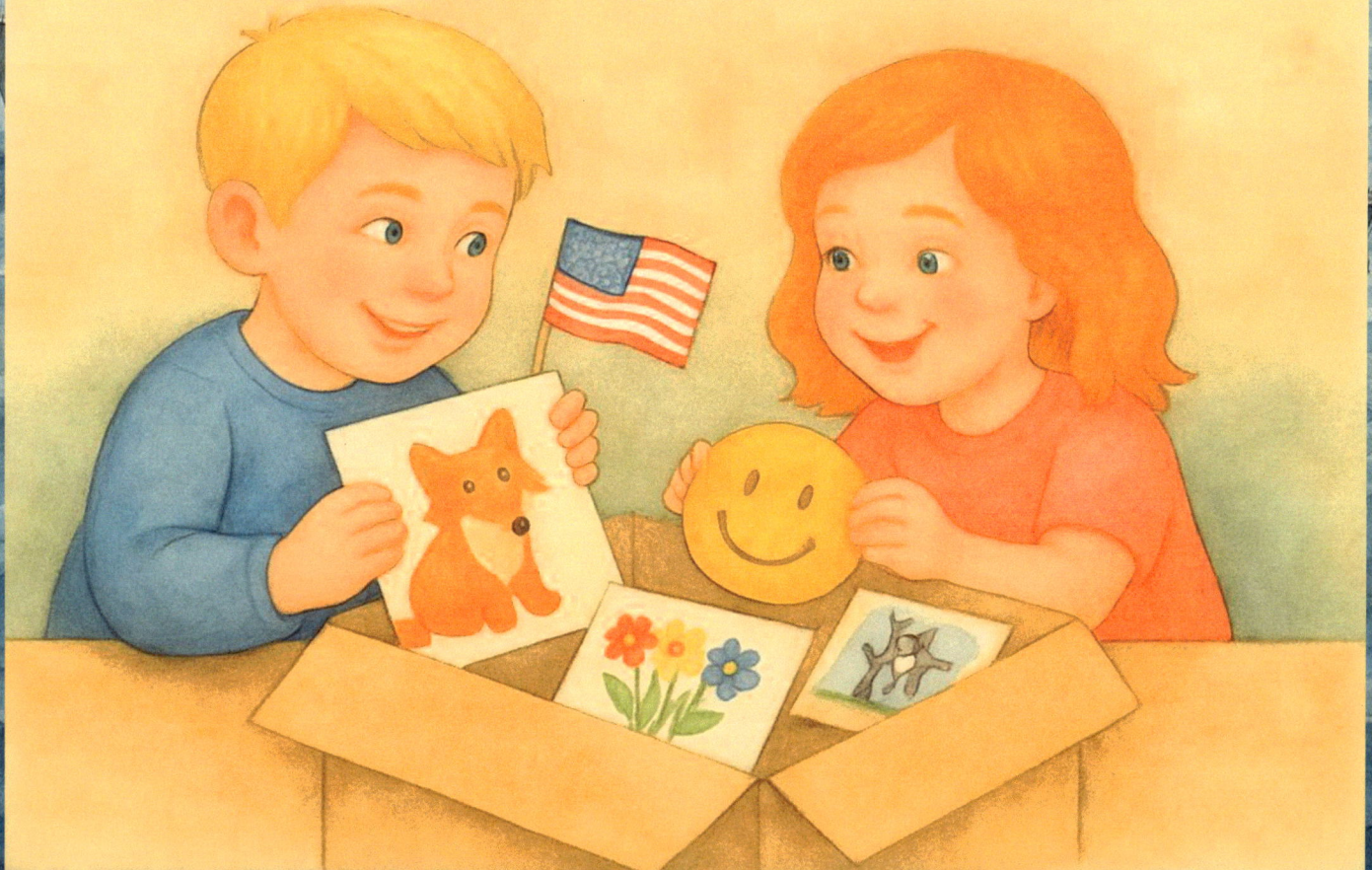

At night, I hug my Daddy doll tight,
It feels like his hug-warm and just right.
I watch his videos—he reads and he smiles,
It's like he's right here, even across miles!

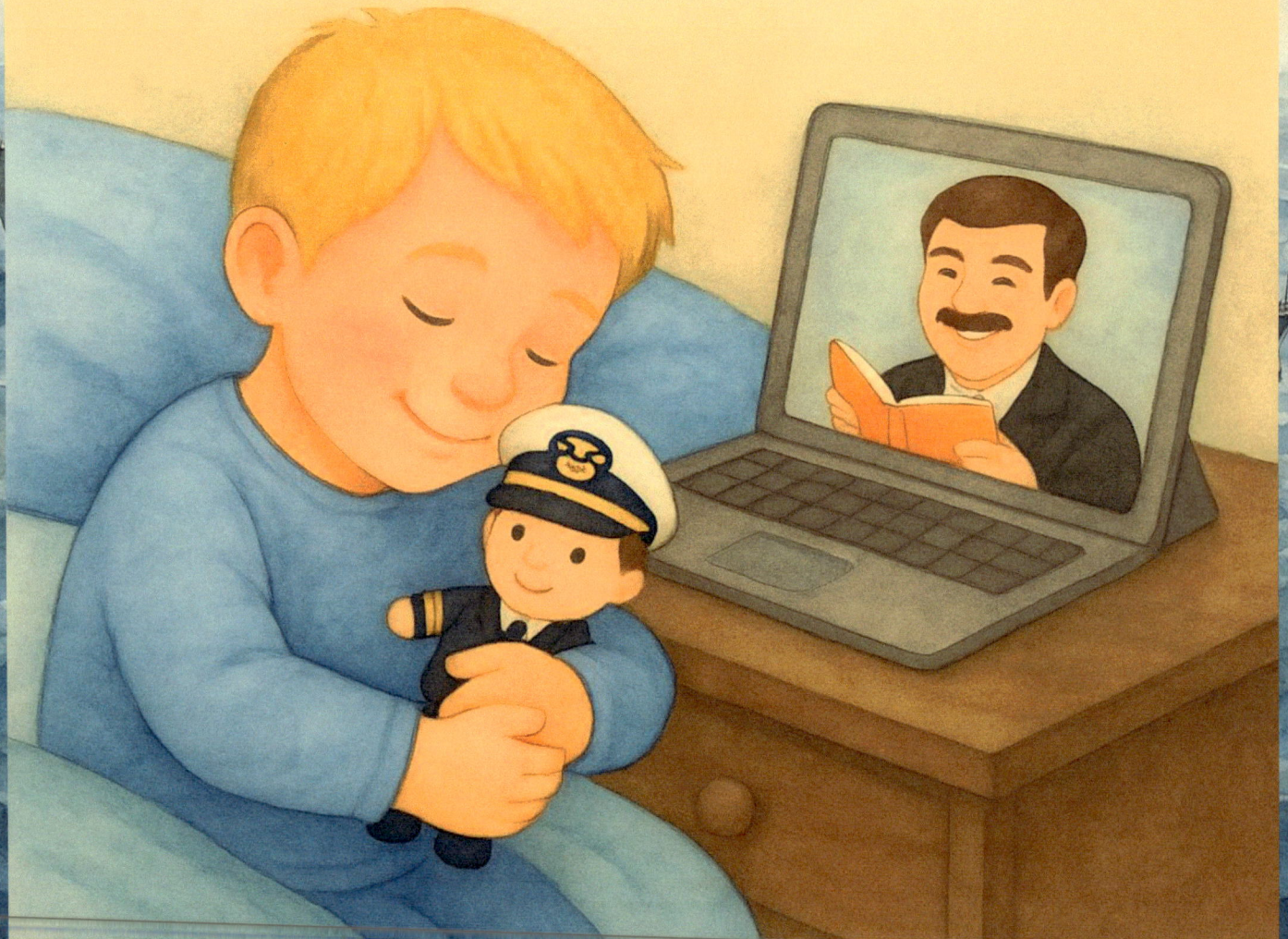

Mommy says it's getting near—
Homecoming day is almost here
That's when Daddy and sailors all come,
Marching back with a great big drum.
We make signs with glitter
and glue, 'Welcome Home!'
in red and blue.

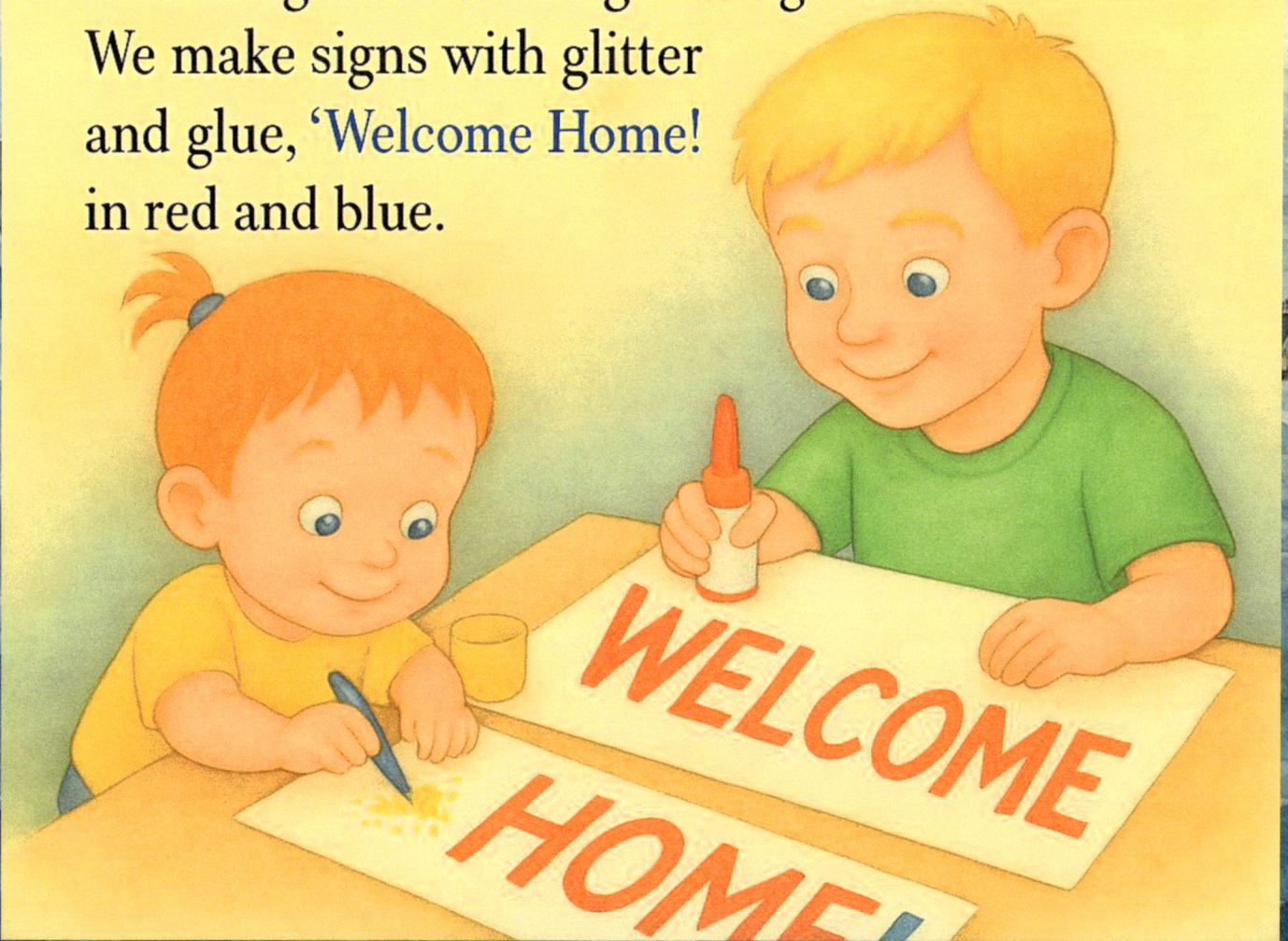

Then—POOF!—the day comes at last,
I put on my best outfit (brand new and fast!).
I wait at the pier with my sign held up high,
Then Dad's here!
I try not to trip on my super–fast feet,
But sometimes I stumble—oops!—
right into his arms.
We laugh and we hug,
and I feel so grand,
The best thing ever—Dad's back
on land!

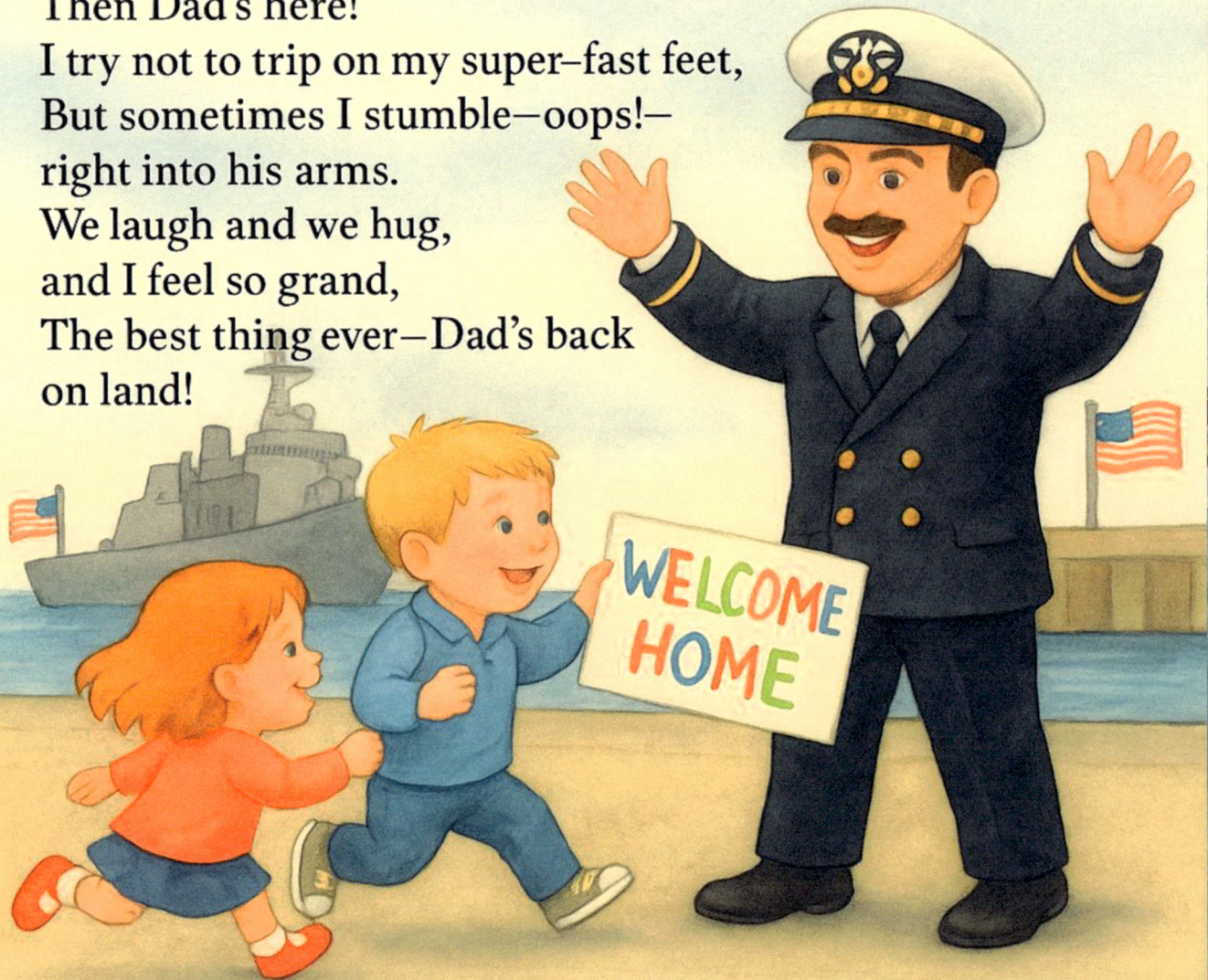

Now Daddy's back home—hooray, hooray!
But guess what? It feels a bit funny today.
He needs some time, and so do I,
We're like two silly fish learning to swim side by side.
We'll get back to us, just give it a few—
With giggles, hugs, and maybe some glue!

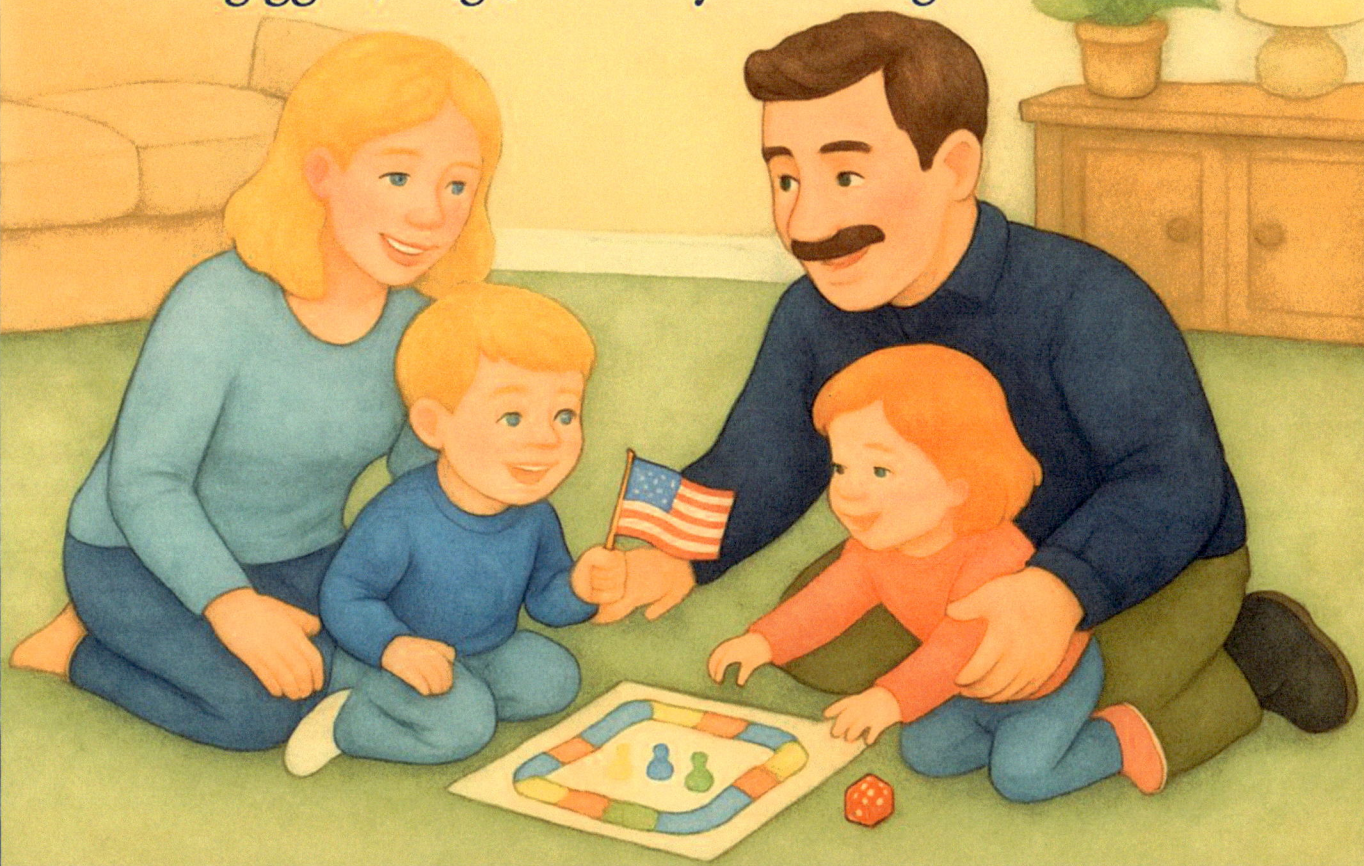

We try to dance but step on each other's toes,
I wear his big boots, and he wears my pink clothes!
We mix up our words and forget what to say,
Like, 'Pass the spaghetti!!' or 'Hide-and-go-play!'
But every day gets a little less weird,
With more silly smiles
and less feeling feared.

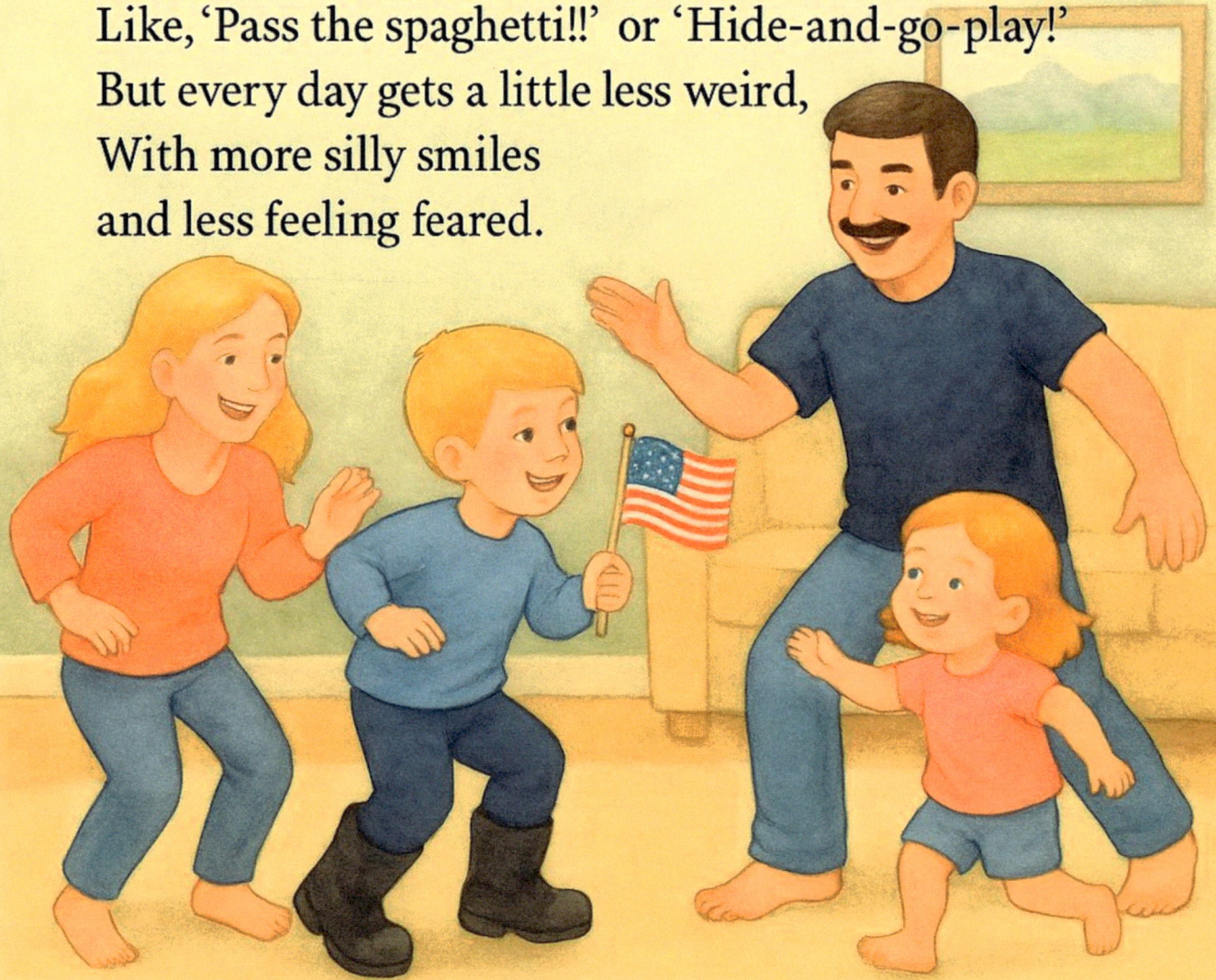

We call it our Gentle Reconnect,
A silly time when we all recollect.
Pancakes stacked high (sometimes way too tall),
And board games where someone always takes a fall!
We laugh, we play, with smiles so wide,
'Cause family's the best wild, wobbly ride!

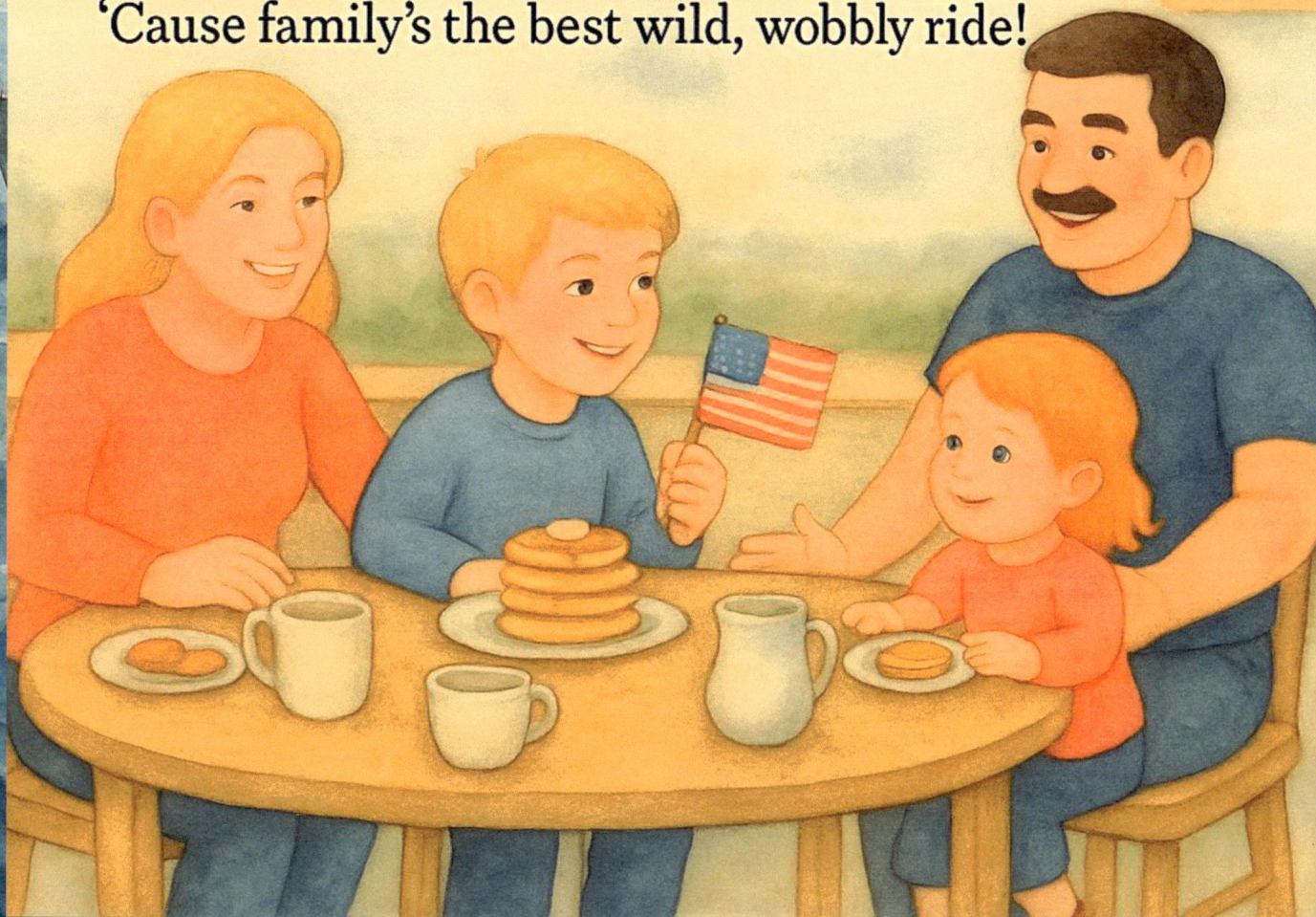

Daddy says love is stretchy and wide,
Like an invisible string we all hold inside.
Whether he's here, or there, or gone for a while—
Our love stays strong, with a big, happy smile!

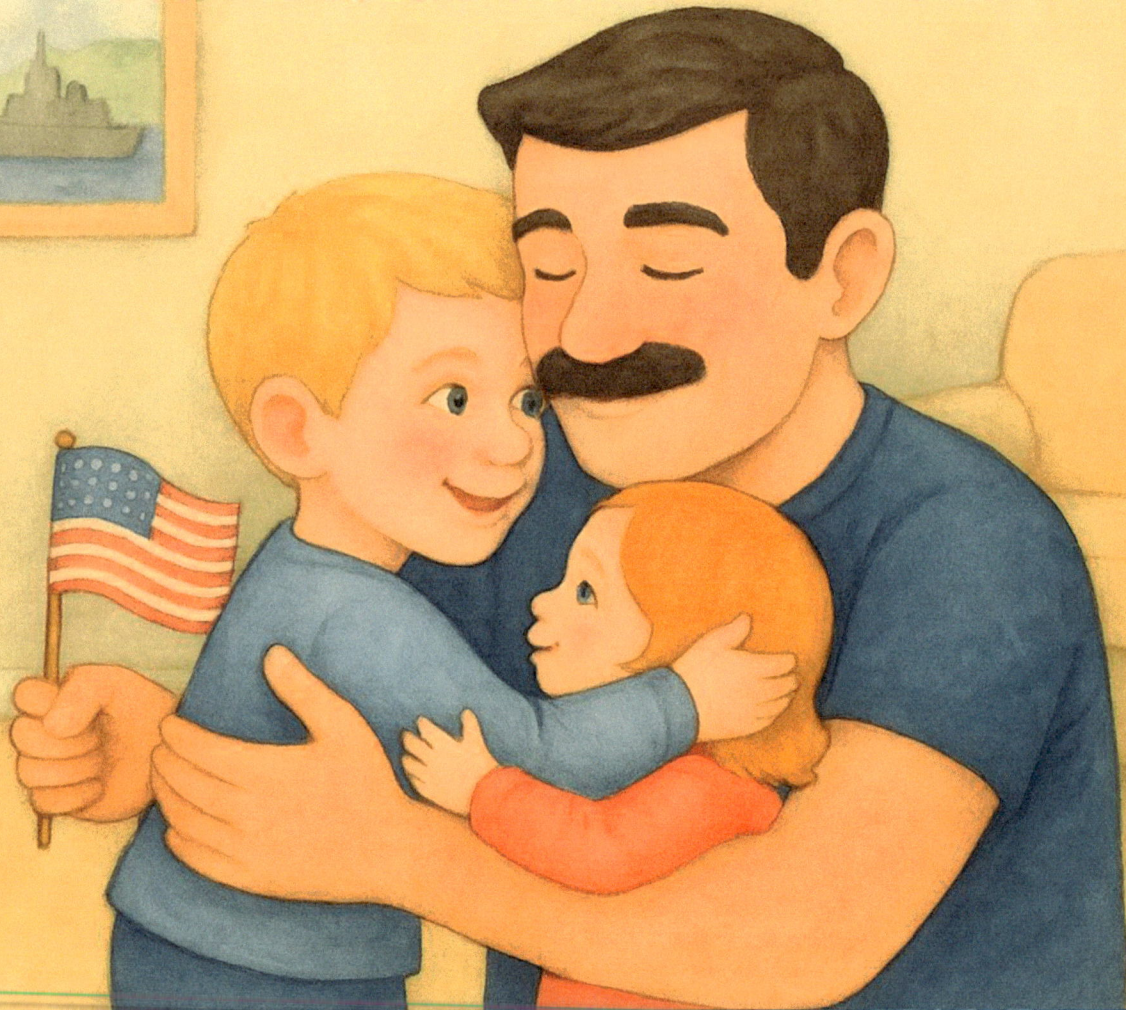

I used to think grown-ups were tough as can be,
But now I'm not sure—that might just be me.
'Cause kids like me? We're made of strong stuff,
Even when days feel heavy and rough.

When people say, 'You must miss him a ton.'
I smile and nod, 'Yeah—but I'm not done.
I'm brave, I'm strong, I carry on too.'

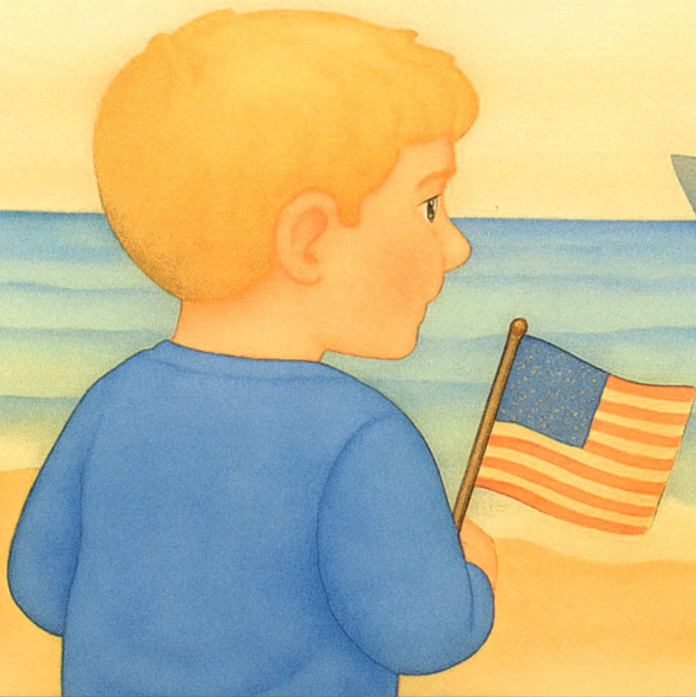

So if your grown-up has to roam,
And you feel a little all alone...
Just talk it out, or dance, or play—
Let your heart sing loud today

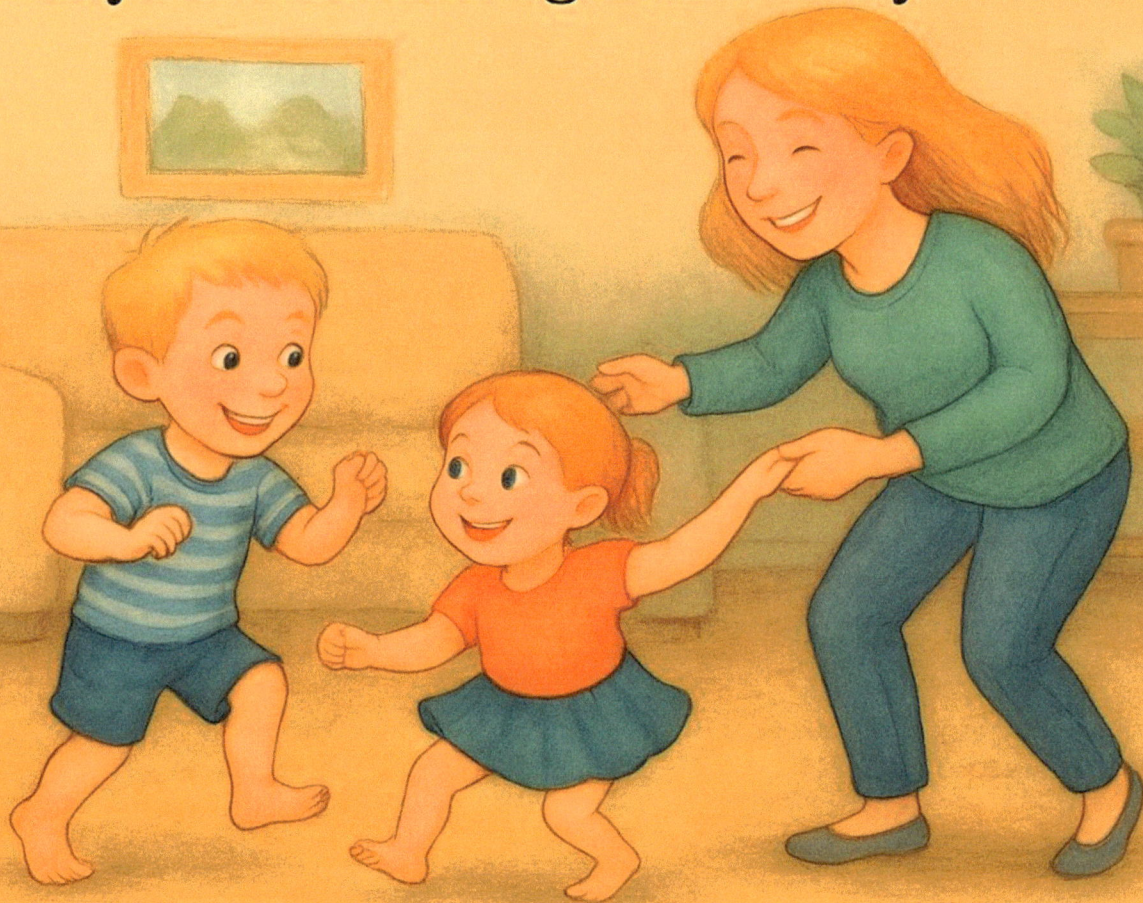

Because even when you're sad or mad,
Or feeling kind of squiggly-bad,
You're never alone—that's the key—
You're strong, you're loved, and brave like me!

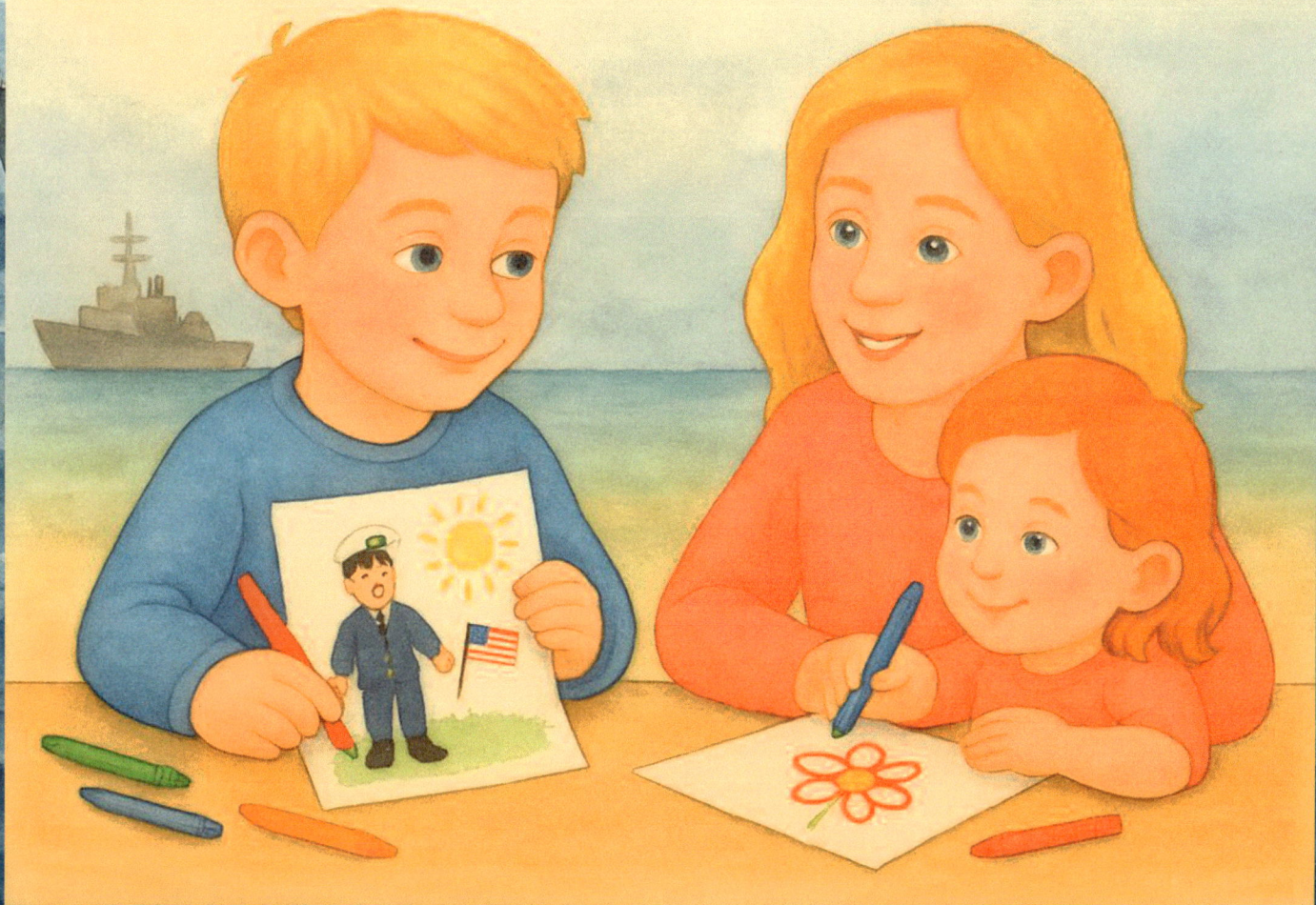

Remember,
Deployment can seem scary and new,
But the moon and the sun shine for both
me and you.
We'll get back to us, just give it a few—
With giggles, hugs, and maybe a few
tears.
Because you're strong,
you're loved, and you
shine bright like me—
A hero in your
own story.

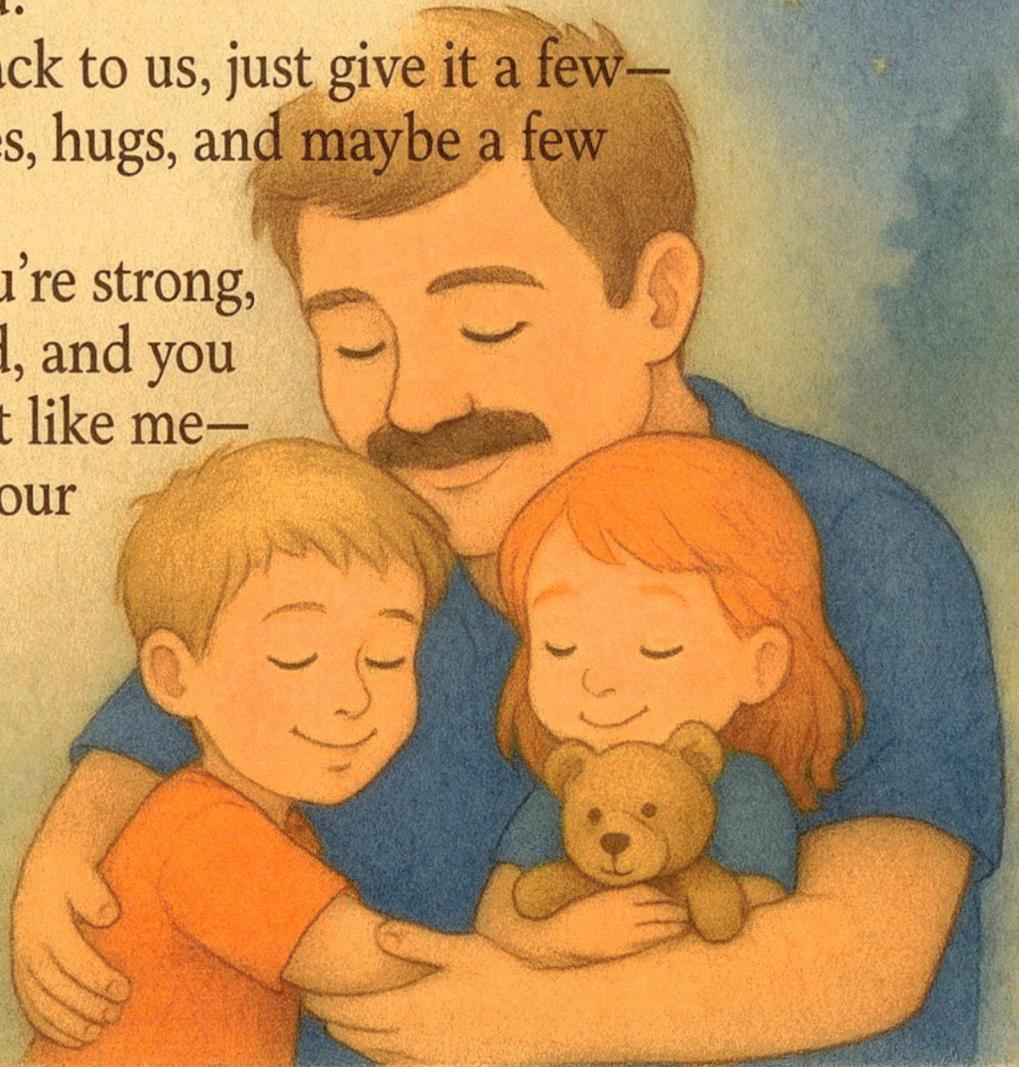

Extra Resources

Blossoming Families

Military Spouse Advocacy Network

Military One Source

National Military Family Association

Military Child Education Coalition

Military Family Advisory Network

Operation Homefront

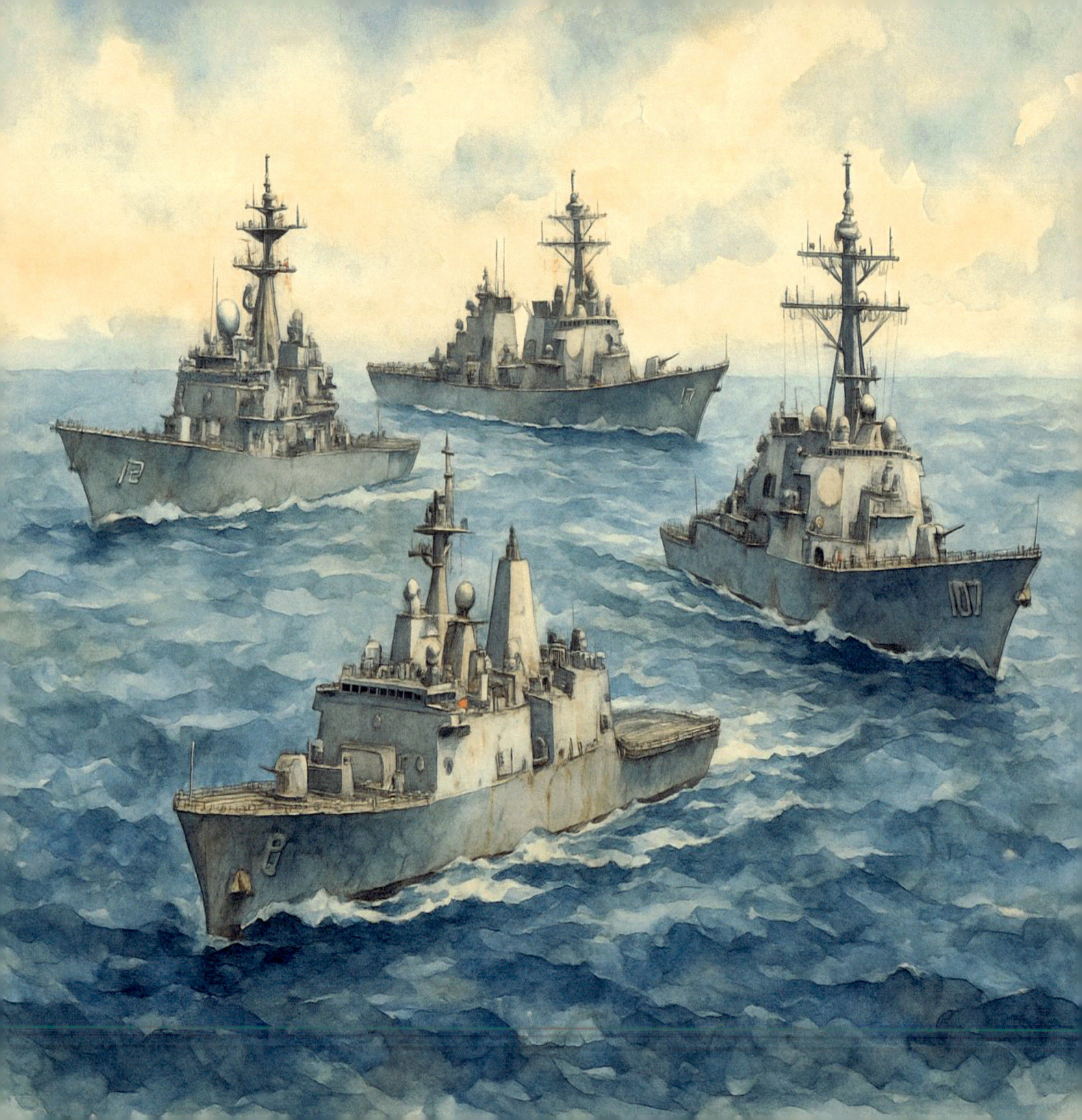

Your Author

Hi! I'm Julia—wife, mom, military spouse, and lifelong advocate for families and children. Military life has brought its fair share of tears, laughter, cross-Atlantic moves, and everything in between. But through it all, I've had the privilege of meeting some truly inspiring people who continue to challenge and motivate me to grow.

My journey as a military spouse led me to pursue a Doctorate in Developmental Psychology. Why? Because I wanted real tools—not just for myself, but to help other military families not just get by, but truly thrive, even when life feels like an uphill climb.

If you're looking for practical ways to strengthen your parenting, boost communication, and build deeper connections, check out my book: *Elevate Yourself: A Roadmap to Having Better Connections*. It's available on Amazon and packed with insights to help you create stronger, happier relationships—at home and beyond.

Here's to lifting each other up!

BLOSSOMING
Families

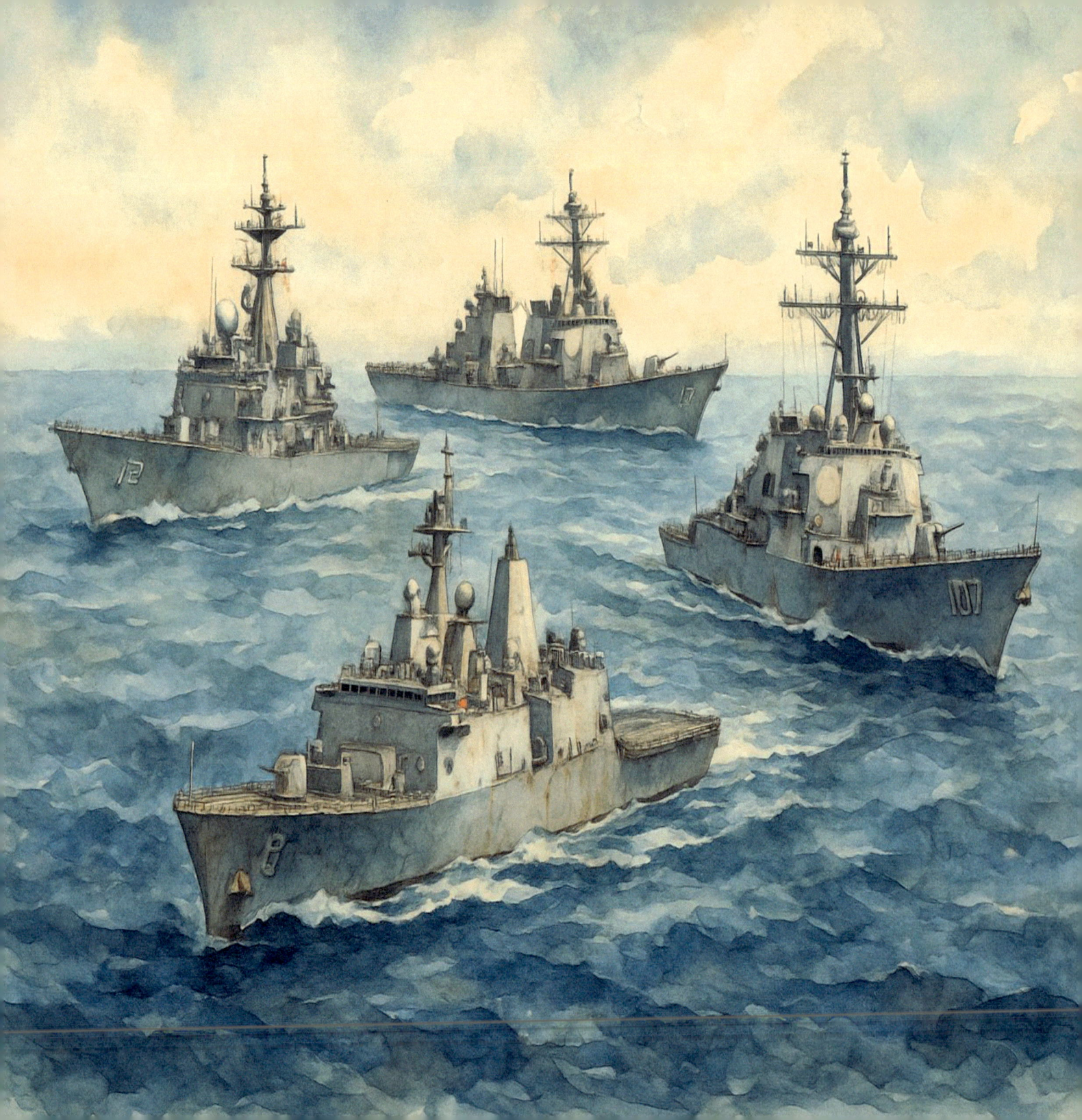

Made in United States
Cleveland, OH
21 June 2025